Selective Laser Trabeculoplasty in Chinese Eyes

Jacky W.Y. Lee
Mandy O.M. Wong
Jason Cheng
Jimmy S.M. Lai

Published by iConcept Press Limited

Published by iConcept Press Limited

Copyright © iConcept Press 2016

http://www.iconceptpress.com

ISBN: 978-1-922227-348

Printed in the United States of America

Contents

Preface

The following book contains a collection of medical research involving the use of Selective Laser Trabeculoplasty (SLT) in the treatment of glaucoma for a Chinese population. As the outcome of glaucoma laser and surgery can have variations among different ethnicities, this book serves to provide Ophthalmic surgeons treating Asian patients, with an evidence based and simple reference guide to maximize the potential of SLT. Much of the research detailed in the book was conducted in Hong Kong over a span of 10 years.

This book touches upon all the fundamentals of the SLT technology from history, laser technique, efficacy in glaucoma subtypes, safely, outcome predictors, to lastly an exploration into the future of laser trabeculoplasty. The book is user-friendly and categorized for a smooth continuous read or as a quick reference guide to particular elements of SLT.

I would like to thank the 3 people who were most instrumental in my journey in Ophthalmology: Dr. Doris W.F. Yick, Dr. Can Y.F. Yuen, and Professor Jimmy S.M. Lai. Their inspirations, training, and mentorship have given life to this book.

This book is dedicated to my parents.

Jacky Lee

The Department of Ophthalmology, Caritas Medical Centre, Hong Kong, China
The Department of Ophthalmology, The University of Hong Kong, China
Dr. Dennis Lam & Partners Eye Center, Hong Kong, China

Author Biography

Jacky W.Y. Lee *FRCOphth, FHKAM (Ophthalmology), FCOphth HK, FRCSEd (Ophth), MRCSEd, MBBS (HK)*

Dr. Lee is a Partner Ophthalmologist at Dennis Lam & Partners Eye Center and Honorary Clinical Assistant Professor at both medical universities in Hong Kong: The University of Hong Kong as well as the Chinese University of Hong Kong. He has 70 publications in peer-reviewed journals and authored 10 book chapters in Ophthalmology. He is the Section Academic Editor of Medicine® and Editorial Board Member of the Asia Pacific Journal of Ophthalmology, International Journal of Ophthalmology, and Hong Kong Journal of Ophthalmology. Dr. Lee serves as a reviewer for 27 international medical journals including The Lancet. Dr. Lee was one of the World Champions in the International Council of Ophthalmology knowledge competition. He has delivered invited lectures, instruction courses, and chaired symposium sessions in a number of international conferences and has served as an examiner for various medical institutions. Dr. Lee was one of the first Ophthalmologists in Hong Kong to introduce the use of the Trabectome® and MicroPulse Laser Trabeculoplasty for Chinese glaucoma patients in Hong Kong.

Mandy O.M. Wong

Dr. Mandy Wong obtained her medical degree (MBBS) at the University of Hong Kong in 2008, and started her ophthalmic training in Hong Kong since 2009. Subsequently, she obtained her postgraduate degree of Master of Public Health at her alma mater in 2013, during which she was awarded the Professor Anthony Hedley Prize in Public Health. She currently works as a specialist ophthalmologist at Hong Kong Eye Hospital(HKEH), and honorary clinical tutor at Department of Ophthalmology and Visual Sciences, the Chinese University of Hong Kong(CUHK). She undertook glaucoma training under the Chinese University of Hong Kong(CUHK)-HKEH Subspecialty Fellowship Program.

Jason Cheng *MBBS BSc FRCOphth, FEBO, FAMS, FRANZCO*

Dr Jason Cheng is a consultant with a special interest in glaucoma and cataract surgery currently working in Singapore. He graduated from Imperial College School of Medicine in the United Kingdom. Following basic medical training in Sydney, Australia, he underwent a 7-year ophthalmology training programme in England which included Moorfields Eye Hospital. He underwent further subspecialty glaucoma training at St Thomas and Kings College London and was awarded a scholarship from the Royal College of Ophthalmologists and Ethicon Foundation fund to complete a second glaucoma fellowship at the University of Toronto. Dr. Cheng is a fellow of the Ophthalmology Colleges of London, Singapore, Australia and New Zealand. He has received multiple awards from various organizations including the Canadian ophthalmology society, Royal College of Ophthalmologist, European board of ophthalmology, National University of Singapore, Singapore Ministry of Health and Imperial College London. He has been awarded 9 research grants, co-authored 11 book chapters, published in respected peer-review medical journals and presented at international conferences.

Jimmy S.M. Lai

Professor Lai graduated at the University of Hong Kong in 1983. Professor Lai received his pre-fellowship training in the Princess Alexandra Eye Pavilion, Edinburgh and post-fellowship training in the Massachusetts Eye and Ear Infirmary, Boston, and the Aichi University, Nagoya, Japan. Professor Lai is currently the Acting Head of the Department of Ophthalmology at the University of Hong Kong, Chief of Service of the Department of Ophthalmology, Queen Mary Hosiptal and Hong Kong University-Shenzhen Hospital, Honorary Director of the Glaucoma Department at the Tianjin Eye Hospital, visiting professor at the Nankai University Eye Hospital, Honorary Professor of the Department of Ophthalmology and Visual Sciences, the Chinese University of Hong Kong, visiting lecturer of the

School of Optometry, the Polytechnic University of Hong Kong. He was the Editor-in-Chief of the Hong Kong Journal of Ophthalmology in 2003-2005 and 2013-2015 and is now the Vice President of the Hong Kong College of Ophthalmologists. He is also member of the editorial board of the Asian Journal of Ophthalmology, Graefe's Archives for Clinical and Experimental Ophthalmology, Journal of Ophthalmology and Research Ophthalmology. Professor Lai is the executive member of the Asian Foundation for the Prevention of Blindness and Honorary Consultant of the Hong Kong Glaucoma patient Association. He serves on the National Medical Research Council (NMRC) International Expert Panel, Ministry of Health, Singapore and Grant Review Board, Health and Medical Research Grant, Hong Kong. He was granted the Distinguished Service Award by the Asian-Pacific Academy of Ophthalmology in 2005 and De Ocampo Award in 2016.

1

Background

The earliest form of laser trabeculoplasty was the Argon Laser Trabeculoplasty (ALT) first introduced in 1979 by Wise and Witter for the treatment of primary open angle glaucoma patients that had high pressures despite medications. Clinical trials soon confirmed the efficacy of ALT as being equivalent to topical medications but the technology was limited by its scar formation tendency and the introduction of more effective prostaglandin eye drops. Following the introduction of selective laser trabeculoplasty (SLT) which offered a safer, scar-free, and seemingly equivalent efficacy, the interest in laser trabeculoplasty has risen again over the years and a number of clinical trials comparing ALT, SLT, and medications have broadened our understanding of this technology.[1]

Factors that may influence the outcome of laser trabeculoplasty include: the degree of angle opening, trabecular meshwork (TM) pigmentation, ethnicity, type of glaucoma, and intraocular pressure (IOP) on presentation. Chinese ethnicity has a greater tendency for angle closure configuration and even in those with open-angle configuration, the access to the TM for angle surgery or laser is often more limited than Caucasian counterparts. The more pigmented TM while in theory allows a greater absorption of laser energy by the pigmented melanocytes, the potential release of iris pigments during laser may however, lead to more IOP spikes post-laser. Furthermore, the narrower the trabecular-iris angle, the closer the proximity of the corneal endothelium to the TM, thus, laser heat dissipation may in theory cause more damage in those with more narrow angles. The incidence of different glaucoma subtypes also varies among different regions and ethnicities and the responses to laser trabeculoplasty will also vary accordingly. Thus, in those of these potential variables, the following chapters will analyze the efficacy and safety of selective laser trabeculoplasty (SLT) based on evidence from the literature that particularly focuses on the Chinese population.

2

History of Selective Laser Trabeculoplasty (SLT)

2.1 History of Selective Laser Trabeculoplasty

Laser trabeculoplasty describes the application of laser on the trabecular meshwork (TM) to achieve lowering of intraocular pressure (IOP). The use of laser on the anterior chamber angle was first introduced in 1961.[2] Researchers including Krasnov[3] and Worthen[4], reported on the decrease in IOP with 'trabeculotomy' or 'laseropuncture'. The effect was, however, not long lasting. In 1979, Wise and Witter introduced the concept of applying argon laser to the trabecular meshwork to 'increase its tension', and achieved IOP control for more than 1 year.[5] The efficacy of argon laser trabeculoplasty (ALT) was further confirmed in the Glaucoma Laser Trial.[6] The application of argon laser to the trabeculum, however, was shown to induce scarring of trabecular meshwork.[7]

In 1995, Latina *et al.* reported on the use of a low energy, q-switched, frequency doubled Nd:Yag laser at a wavelength of 532 nm and pulse duration of 3 to 10 nanoseconds in performing laser trabeculoplasty.[8] It was shown that selective targeting of pigmented trabecular meshwork cells could be achieved with this laser, sparing the adjacent non-pigmented trabecular meshwork cells from collateral thermal or structural damage.[8] In 1998, Latina *et al.*[9] published on the success of selective laser trabeculoplasty (SLT) in reducing IOP by 23.5% in patients with uncontrolled open angle glaucoma (OAG), and 24.2% in patients with uncontrolled OAG previously treated with ALT. Since then, SLT has gained increasing attention as a potentially repeatable treatment for OAG patients. The reported efficacy of SLT in lowering IOP ranged from 11 to 40%.[10]

2.2   Mechanism of Selective Laser Trabeculoplasty

Several mechanisms were postulated to explain the IOP lowering effect of laser trabeculoplasty. The mechanical effect of laser was demonstrated with morphological and histological studies.[7, 11] In monkeys receiving ALT, scarring was seen to obliterate TM in spots treated with laser.[11] The mechanical theory postulated that the mechanical effect caused an decrease in the circumference of the trabecular ring by tissue shrinkage, pulling open the intertrabecular spaces and increasing the outflow facility.[5] An alternative explanation by Van der Zypen was the widening of intertrabecular spaces secondary to the contraction of adjacent treated areas.[12] This theory, however, did not fully explain the effect of laser trabeculoplasty. For example, there was no difference in the area of Schlemm's canal after ALT.[13] The mechanical effect of laser seemed to be more prominent in eyes treated with ALT, but much less in those treated with SLT.[7] Alternative theories were postulated to explain the effect of laser trabeculoplasty.

In addition to the mechanical theory, cellular and biologic mechanisms were proposed to explain the reduction of IOP post trabeculoplasty through a cascade of cytokine up-regulation, phacocytic activity and repopulation of the TM.[10] Bradley *et al.* demonstrated up-regulation of interleukin-1 and tumor necrosis factor-α, which may in turn stimulate trabecular matrix metalloproteinase expression and juxtacanalicular extracellular matrix remodeling that decreased the outflow resistance from the eye.[14, 15] Another hypothesis on increased cell division and TM repopulation was supported by in-vitro studies by the group of Bylsma *et al.*, which showed 180% increase in the basal level of DNA replication in the 2 days immediately after ALT[16], and a four-fold increase in cell division over untreated controls.[17] As little mechanical damage was shown in SLT treated areas of TM as compared to those treated with ALT[7], mechanism of SLT was believed to be more biological than mechanical.[10]

2.3   Efficacy of SLT

The application of SLT had been reported in various types of OAG, including primary open angle glaucoma (POAG), pseudoexfoliation glaucoma (PEX), pigment dispersion syndrome (PDS), normal tension glaucoma (NTG) and ocular hypertension (OHT). Most recently, a few studies were carried out to investigate the efficacy of SLT in angle closure disease.[18, 19] Until 2013, efficacy of SLT in lower IOP in OAG was shown in more than 30 studies.[20-54]

2.4   Comparison to Argon Laser Trabeculoplasty (ALT)

Several randomised controlled trials were performed to compare the efficacy of SLT with ALT.[23, 37, 44, 55] All except one study by Rosenfeld et al.[44] were performed in Canada, with the latter one performed in Israel. The ethnicity of patients included Asian, black and white in the study by Liu et al., 2012[37], but ethnicity of subjects was not mentioned in the other studies. Various types of OAG, including POAG, juvenile OAG, PEX, PDS, OHT, NTG and mixed mechanism glaucoma were included. Patients selected were on medication in the study by Liu et al., 2012[37], and had uncontrolled OAG despite maximally tolerated medication or previous ALT in the rest of the studies, with mean baseline IOP of 19.1 to 25.4 mmHg.

The power of SLT used in these studies spanned from 0.47 to 1.5 mJ, or total power of 31.9 ± 29.4 mJ, with application over 180 to 360° of TM. Duration of studies ranged from 6 months to 5 years. Definition of treatment success was different across studies, including IOP reduction of 15 to 20% or ≥ 3 mmHg, and without additional need for further interventions for IOP control. Two of the studies reported also the reduction of number of medication.[23, 37]

Results of the SLT arms of these studies showed a mean IOP reduction of 7.7 to 31.1% from baseline, and treatment success of 25 to 75%. Among these studies, Bovell et al.[23] reported on the longest follow-up period of 5 years post laser trabeculoplasty with the largest sample size of 89 eyes in the SLT arm. While both SLT and ALT arms showed statistically insignificant difference in reduction of IOP over 5 years, in those with previous ALT ≥ 360°, the SLT group showed a statistically insignificant superiority of 5.9 mmHg in IOP reduction compared to ALT. The success rate was also similar between both arms throughout the follow-up period, with the success rate of SLT being 44% at 3 years, 38% at 4 years and 25% at 5 years.

In a meta-analysis on the comparison of efficacy of SLT versus ALT[56], there was no significant difference in the pooled mean reduction in IOP, reduction in medication, and treatment success between the 2 groups, showing non-inferiority of SLT compared to ALT in IOP lowering in OAG patients.

2.5   Comparison to Anti-glaucoma Medications

With the advent of potent IOP lowering medication in recent decades, comparison of SLT to anti-glaucoma medication is crucial in identifying the position of SLT in the treatment algorithm of OAG.

Several randomised controlled trials reported on the efficacy of SLT versus medication.[33, 36, 57, 58] The studies were carried out in the United States, Hong Kong, and United Kingdom respectively, including different ethnicities including Caucasian, Chinese and African patients. All patients were OAG patients and were not on any concomitant medication for the eyes receiving treatment. In particular, the study by Lai *et al.*[36] used fellow eyes that received topical medications only, as a control. IOP-lowering medication in various combinations were used in the control arms in 2 studies[33, 36], while latanoprost 0.005% was used in the studies by Nagar *et al.*[57, 58] The mean baseline IOP in the SLT arm ranged from 25.0 to 26.8 mmHg.

The power of SLT used in these studies ranged from 0.2 to 1.7 mJ, treating 180 to 360° of the TM. Duration of the studies ranged from 4 – 6 months to 5 years. Definition of treatment success varied among studies, including no additional need for SLT as assessed by individual target IOP and visual field assessment, IOP < 21mmHg with or without maximal medication, or IOP reduction ≥ 20%.

The reduction of IOP in the SLT group ranged from 18.0 to 32.1%, with treatment success rate from 65 to 89%. Of note, the design of the study by Katz *et al.*[33] allowed comparison of SLT treatment with medication use and the SLT arm had repeated SLT treatments in case of initial treatment failure. It showed comparable reduction in IOP between the 2 groups at last follow-up (26.4% in the SLT group versus 27.8% in the medical group). However, it also demonstrated a higher need for stepping up of treatment for IOP control in the medical arm versus the SLT arm (27% versus 11%) at 9 to 12 months follow-up. While this study showed the results up to 1 year, the other study by Lai *et al.*[36] compared the effect of SLT and medication over 5 years. Eyes that had inadequate IOP control despite SLT were allowed to use additional medical therapy. The study showed a comparable mean IOP reduction over 5 years between both arms, with a significantly lower mean number of medications in the SLT group.

In comparing the pooled effect of IOP reduction and treatment success of SLT with the medication group among the available randomized controlled trials in our meta-analysis[56], medication group achieved a reduction of 0.85 mmHg more than the SLT group. The odds ratio of SLT group achieving success compared to medication was 0.8, showing a possible advantage in medical therapy. However, these differences were not statistically significant.

3

The Use SLT in Different Glaucoma Subtype

The mainstream primary treatment for glaucoma is still currently using anti-glaucoma eye drops to lower the IOP. Unfortunately, these eye drops contain both local and systemic side effects including conjunctival injection, allergic conjunctivitis, hypertrichiasis, iris pigmentations, cystoids macular edema, bradycardia, and bronchospasms. Multiple medications may be required to achieve adequate IOP control especially in those with rapid disease progression, further adding to the side effects and inconveniences of medication use. In the past, various interventions have been implemented to encourage anti-glaucoma drug adherence including the use of simplified regimes, reminder devices, as well as education and individualized care planning[59] but what is really needed for glaucoma patients is a treatment option that will inflict minimal interference to patients' daily activities whilst achieving effective IOP lowering.

3.1 Primary-open Angle Glaucoma (POAG)

In POAG, the findings from the Early Manifest Glaucoma Trial[60] and the Advanced Glaucoma Intervention Study[61] suggested than an IOP reduction of more than 25% from presentation and an IOP control less than 18 mmHg respectively would reduce the chance of disease progression. In theory, SLT should be effective in pigmented eyes as the laser selectively targets melanocytes. However, in Chinese eyes, this is often offset by the fact that even in eyes that meet the angle classification of POAG (≥ 270° of visible anterior TM), the pigmented TM but not always be fully accessible especially in phakic patients. In Chapter 1, we have established that SLT is as effective as topical anti-glaucoma medications and ALT but without the topical side effects of medications and without the coagulative damage and scarring of ALT. Lee *et al.* reported in a randomized control trial comparing SLT with medication that at 6 months, the SLT group had a 7.6% lower IOP and required 40.0% less medication compared to the medical group. Both the SLT (40.9%) and the medication only group (41.9%) achieved a similar percentage of IOP reduction compared to their IOP on first presentation.[62] Lai *et al.* reported in their randomized control trial that at 5 years after SLT, the SLT group had a mean IOP decreased by 32% (from 26.8 mmHg to 18.3 mmHg) but there was no statistical difference in IOP reduction compared to the control group that received topical medications alone although the SLT group required fewer medications to maintain IOP < 21 mmHg (P < 0.001). Only 27.6% of patients in SLT group required medications to control IOP < 21 mmHg at 5 years. The failure rate, which was defined as an IOP > 21 mmHg with maximal medications was 17.2% in the SLT group versus 27.6% in medication group (P = 0.53). Around 10.3% of treated eyes had a transient post-SLT IOP spike > 5 mmHg within the first day after SLT.[36] Thus, SLT is an effective alternative to medication for IOP control with demonstrated sustainability for up to 5 years in some patients. Overall, the requirement for medication is lower than using medication alone to achieve the same degree of IOP control.

3.2   Primary Angle-closure Glaucoma (PACG)

PACG is characterized by angle configuration of ≥ 270° of grade 0 – 1 on the Shaffer grading in the presence of glaucomatous optic neuropathy. Ho *et al.* investigated 60 patients who had PACG with IOP > 21 mmHg, a patent laser iridotomy, and a gonioscopically visible pigmented TM > 90°. SLT was performed to the 90° of open-angle area and at 6 months, the IOP lowering response was as follow: 82% > 3 mmHg reduction, 72% > 4 mmHg reduction, 54% ≥ 20% IOP reduction, and 24% ≥ 30% IOP reduction. The mean IOP decreased by 24% in 6 months (from 24.6 mmHg to 18.7mmHg).[19] More recently, in a randomized control trial by Narayanaswamy *et al.*, in 100 subjects with primary angle closure (PAC) or PACG subjects with 180° of visible posterior TM on gonioscopy, 50 received SLT and 50 received travoprost 0.004% for IOP control. At 6 months, both groups had a statistically similar percent of IOP reduction (16.9% versus 18.5%, P = 0.52) while complete success (IOP ≤ 21 mmHg without medications) was 60.0% in SLT group and 84.0% in the medication group (P = 0.008). One patient in the SLT group (2.0%) had a transient post-treatment IOP spike > 5 mm Hg. In the short-term, SLT was effective in IOP reduction for PAC or PACG but more long-term evaluation is currently not available in the literature.

3.3   Normal Tension Glaucoma (NTG)

NTG is a type of open angle glaucoma with glaucomatous optic nerve damage but intraocular pressure (IOP) that never exceeds 21 mmHg.[63] NTG has a high prevalence in Asia, accounting for 77 and 92% of the POAG cases in Korea and Japan respectively.[64, 65] The Collaborative Normal Tension Glaucoma Study has shown that a 30% reduction in IOP can slow the progression of NTG and IOP fluctuation has also been demonstrated to contribute to NTG progression.[66, 67] It is often difficult for NTG patients to fully understand the need for regular anti-glaucoma medications as their IOP is told to be "within normal range" on every clinical visit and they are symptom free until very late in their disease. The side effects (redness, dry eyes, allergies) from topical anti-glaucoma medications are often the only symptoms experienced by NTG patients.

As early as the 1980's, ALT was used to successfully treat NTG, achieving IOP reductions of 4.9 mmHg at 12 months with a gradual tapering of the pressure-lowering effect over the course of a 21.6-month follow-up.[68] The trabecular scarring and destructive nature of ALT limited its clinical practicality for those who lost the pressure-lowering effective with time.

Literature on the use of SLT for NTG is scanty, with reported IOP reductions ranging from 12 to 15% in only a few small case series involving 11 to 18 subjects.[25, 69] In studies that had a mixed population of POAG, NTG, and OHT subjects, the 1-year IOP reduction ranged from 14 to 15%.[69, 70] Lee *et al.* from Hong Kong reported that SLT was effective in lowering the IOP by 20% and 15% at 6 months and 1 year respectively. The number of medication used was also reduced by and 27% at both 6 months and 1 year after laser.[71, 72] Similarly, Nitta *et al.*[41] used SLT as the initial treatment in 42 NTG subjects and reported IOP reductions of 16.5% at 1 year and 14.6% at 2 years. Lee *et al.* reported that at 2 years, the IOP was reduced by 11.5% and medication reduction of around 41.1%.[73]

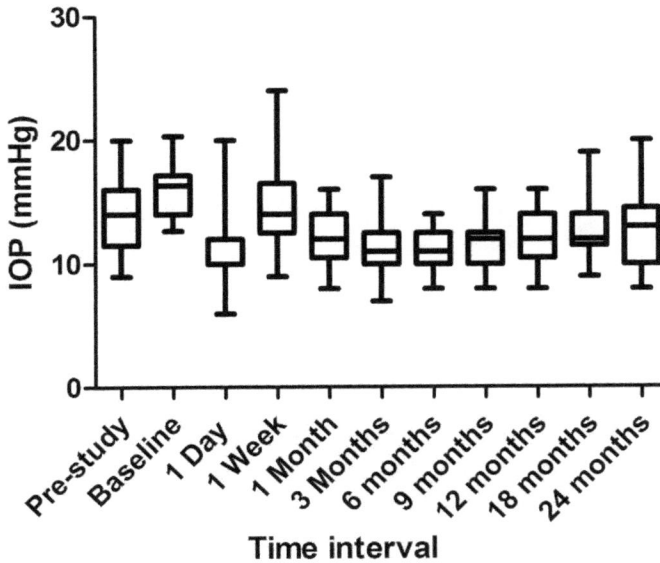

Figure 1: Changes in IOP after SLT for NTG over 24 months[73]

Lee *et al.* also reported a gradual decline in the absolute success (IOP reduction > 20% without medication) of 61% at 6 months to an absolute success of 22% at 12-months, as the effect of SLT is well known to decrease with time but because the laser is non-scarring, it can be repeated.[72] Lee *et al.* reported that at 1 year after SLT, the mean survival rate of the procedure was 95.1%; only 2 subjects required a secondary SLT after the first procedure.[71]

While the IOP reduction of SLT in NTG is inferior to that of POAG or PACG, SLT is still particularly useful in NTG patients because the majority of these patients are asymptomatic and told by their doctors to have "normal" pressures during clinical visits. Thus, issues with drug compliance and medication side effects are magnified in this group of patients who may have more difficulties in understanding the nature of their disease. However, while SLT may partially deal with the IOP component of NTG, the hypoperfusion element of NTG cannot be addressed by laser therapy and systemic optimization of the NTG patient is still required to supplement the effects of SLT.

4

SLT Technique and Optimal Energy

4.1 Preparation

Many gonioscopic lenses can be used for SLT. It is best to contact the developer of your SLT laser system to find a lens that is suitable for use. However, after each use, it is important to highlight that alcohol should not be used to disinfect the SLT lenses since alcohol has been shown to cause superficial keratopathy and corneal edema, which can affect corneal structure and function.[74] Instead, it is more suitable to use disinfecting agents like Presept 0.5 grams disinfection tablets (Johnson & Johnson, New Brunswick, New Jersey 08933, United States of America), which has not been known to cause keratopathy. All lenses should be rinsed with normal saline after disinfection.

Anesthesia can be achieved using the standard topical anesthetic eye drops used for Goldmann applanation tonometry. The majority of patients can tolerate SLT without much discomfort. For those with a lower pain threshold, Xylocaine gel or oral analgesics may be used to achieve analgesia.

The decision to washout medications before SLT treatment is still controversial. In a retrospective study by Scherer,[75] IOP reduction was greatest in POAG subjects being treated with prostaglandin analogues. On the other hand, Alvarado *et al.*[76] found that prostaglandin analogues might limit the efficacy of SLT. Moreover, Singh *et al.*[77] reported no significant difference in SLT success following prostaglandin analogue use.

4.2   Laser Applications

SLT is performed with fixed laser duration of 3 nanoseconds and a spot size of 400 µm. Patients should be treated with an initial energy of 0.8 mJ and the power can be titrated up or down until bubble formation is just visible and titrated to a lower energy level if excessive pain is experienced. The TM should be treated in a 360° fashion as Nagar *et al.* previously reported a higher success rate with 360° treatment (93 – 102 spots) compared to 180° (48 – 53 spots) or 90° (25 – 30 spots) treatment.[58]

A single drop of alpha-adrenergic agonist may be instilled after the procedure to prevent IOP spikes which can occur in up to 10% of subjects within the first 1 – 2 hours after the procedure.[36] The choice of post-laser eye drops is surgeon dependent, ranging from no eye drops to topical non-steroidal eye drops to a weak topical steroid. In principle, the use of an anti-inflammatory agent should be kept to a minimum (weak steroid and short duration of use) to prevent over-suppression of the inflammatory cytokines responsible for biological effects of SLT on the TM.

Subjects should be follow-up on day 1, 1 week, 1 month, and then every 3 – 6 months depending on clinical need.

4.3   Optimizing Outcome

SLT energy has been reported to be one of the factors that influence a successful outcome.[78] A greater span of angle treatment has also been found to improve success. Treatment to 360° of the trabecular meshwork was found to lower IOP as effectively as latanoprost 0.005%, but in those receiving only 90° or 180° treatments, the IOP-lowering efficacy was inferior.[58] Rinke *et al.* likewise reported that 360° of SLT treatment was superior to 180° treatment in 36 eyes with OAG.[79]

However, overlapping laser spots does not seem to further improve outcome. In a retrospective review of 318 open-angle eyes, the use of 100 overlapping SLT spots over 180° resulted in a poorer IOP response than those treated in a non-overlapping fashion over 360°.[80]

Recently, Lee *et al.*[81] postulated that it is not only the absolute number of spots that determine SLT response but rather the total energy density (number of spots multiplied by the mean energy) delivered that is of importance. They investigated in a group of 49 Chinese OAG subjects that received 360° SLT treatment, the optimal interval and point of total SLT energy that resulted in the largest drop in IOP by using Bandwidth selection by generalized cross-validation. The 95% confidence band by bootstrap analysis revealed that at energy intervals between 214.6 to 234.9 mJ, the IOP was significantly decreased by > 25%, with the optimal total energy at 226.1 mJ.

4.4 Post-laser Care

The majority of patients receiving SLT will experience minimal to zero discomfort during the procedure and the post-operative care is relatively straightforward. Some patients may experience a dull eye pain and radiating headache, which may be treated with simple oral analgesics. Topical anti-inflammatory eye drops may not be required as the majority of anterior chamber reactions following SLT are mild and self-limiting within 1 week of laser.[82] Where required, a weak topical steroid for a short frequency and duration or a topical non-steroidal anti-inflammatory agent may be used with the understanding that excessive suppression of the anterior chamber reaction may also inhibit the inflammatory cytokines that are responsible in increasing the permeability of the TM and hence aqueous outflow following SLT.

Patients are usually required to follow-up on day 1 and 1 week following SLT to observe for the potential anterior chamber reaction and potential IOP spikes. The IOP reduction may reach a plateau anywhere between 2 weeks to 3 months but a previous study has demonstrated that the 3 month IOP was correlated with the IOP at 2 and 4 weeks after laser.[83] Thus, by 4 weeks, the anti-glaucoma medications may be adjusted up or down to achieve individual target pressures.

5

Predictors of Success with SLT

Not all treated individuals respond to SLT. It is therefore useful to understand the potential parameters that may influence a successful outcome. It has been reported that treatment in medication naive eyes may result in a greater success[40, 79, 84] and that the use of a prostaglandin eye drop may impair the success to SLT.[47] Other factors including age and the degree of angle pigmentation were inconclusive throughout the literature.[9, 85] Other parameters including diabetes, central corneal thickness, lens status (phakic versus pseudophakic), and angle status were found to be unassociated with SLT success. [86]

Lee *et al.*[87-89] recently published a series on the predictors of success of SLT in a Chinese population among different glaucoma subtypes. They analyzed 25 covariates (including type of glaucoma, phakic status, age, sex, pre and post-treatment IOP, different types of medications, various corneal parameters, visual acuity, laser energy, and disease severity as assessed by visual field and Optical Coherence Tomography) using univariate and multiple logistic regression analyses separately in subjects with OAG, NTG, and POAG independently. The success to SLT is most commonly defined as an IOP reduction by ≥ 3 mmHg[90, 91] or more commonly by an IOP reduction of $\geq 20\%$ while keeping the same number of anti-glaucoma medications.[47, 92]

5.1 Open-angle Glaucoma (OAG)

In 111 eyes of 65 subjects with OAG (60 NTG and 51 POAG), the overall success rate was 53.15%, with a mean IOP reduction of 19.81 ± 15.93%. In both univariate/multivariate analyses, a higher pre-SLT IOP was a significant predictor for success (coefficient = 0.20/0.46, OR = 1.23/1.58, P = 0.0017/0.0011) while using 3 anti-glaucoma medications (coefficient = –1.08/–3.74, OR = 0.3/0.024, P = 0.037/ P = 0.0081) was associated with SLT failure. Hodge and Mao likewise reported an odds ratio of 1.58[93] and 1.3[94], respectively when pre-treatment IOP was used as a predictor of success. Furthermore, every 1 mmHg increase in the pre-treatment IOP resulted in a 30% increase in likelihood for success. [86]

5.2 POAG

In 51 eyes with POAG, the success rate of SLT was 47.1%. The following parameters were associated with greater success using univariate analysis including: older age (coefficient = 0.1, OR = 1.1, P = 0.0003), a higher pre-treatment IOP (coefficient = 0.3, OR = 1.3, P = 0.0005), using 4 types of anti-glaucoma eye drops (coefficient = 2.1, OR = 8.4, P = 0.005), a greater dioptre (D) of spherical equivalent (coefficient = 2.1, OR = 8.4, P = 0.005), and the use of a topical carbonic anhydrase inhibitor (coefficient = 1.7, OR = 6.0, P = 0.003).[87]

Subjects with poorer disease control or higher IOP were more likely to require a greater number of anti-glaucoma medications; hence, the association between the number of medications used may in fact be an indirect association with the pre-treatment IOP. The mean refractive status in the above population was –3.54 ± 4.05 D. Hence, those with a greater dioptre of spherical equivalent were more likely to be more myopic and hence a deeper anterior chamber angle allowing for more accessible areas for SLT treatment. Although in the Caucasian population, angle status was not found to correlate with SLT success, the Chinese population often have a higher prevalence of narrower angles, thus, a deeper anterior chamber with better visualization of the trabecular meshwork is important in Chinese.

5.3 NTG

In 60 eyes with NTG, the success rate of SLT was 61.7%. In multivariate analysis, having a higher pre-treatment IOP (coefficient = 1.1, OR = 3.1, P = 0.05) and a lower 1-week IOP (coefficient = –0.8, OR = 0.5, P = 0.04) were associated with greater SLT success. It is postulated that the release of metalloproteinase, cytokines, and macrophages would be most florid immediately after SLT, therefore, those that have a greater IOP reduction within the first week of laser may signify a greater biochemical response to SLT.

6

Side Effects of SLT

SLT was approval by the United States Food and Drug Administration in 2001 for the treatment of OAG. In contrary to the former ALT, SLT uses only 1% of the energy in ALT and does not result in visible or histological trabecular meshwork scarring.[95] It is generally a very safe procedure with only a few reported transient side effects throughout the literature including: anterior chamber reaction, IOP spikes, eye pain, conjunctivitis, corneal edema, and blurred vision.[9, 40, 96] Permanent corneal damage is extremely rare. Moubayed *et al.* was the first to report a case with permanent corneal edema developing into bullous keratopathy following SLT.[97] There are 2 additional reported cases where corneal edema, haze, and thinning occurred within 24 – 48 hours after SLT resulting in corneal scarring and refractive error changes.[98] One of these cases was tested positive for Herpes Simplex Virus-1, hence herpetic re-activation may have attributed to these changes.[98]

IOP spikes of > 5mmHg can occur within few hours after SLT and may be treated with a drop of alpha-adrenergic agonist before or after the procedure.[36] At 1 week, the IOP may also rise but seldom beyond the pretreatment level; the IOP gradually reaches a plateau from approximately 1 month onwards.[71].

Given the close proximity of the trabecular meshwork to the cornea especially in Chinese that tend to have narrower angles than Caucasians, it is important understand the corneal changes that take place following SLT. Lee *et al.* investigated 111 eyes of 66 Chinese OAG subjects that received SLT. The endothelial cell count via a specular microscopy, central corneal thickness (CCT) via a videokeratography, and spherical equivalent via a kerato-refractometer was measure before and at 1 month after SLT. The intraclass correlation coefficient of these investigations was 0.997, signifying high reproducibility.

The majority of anterior chamber inflammation settle within 3 to 5 days thus, aggressive steroid use should be avoided after SLT in order to excessive suppression of the inflammation cascade which plays a role in the biochemical actions of SLT in reducing the permeability of the outflow pathway.[99]

The mean endothelial cell count significantly decreased by 4.5% from 2465.0 ± 334.0 cells/mm^2 at baseline to 2355.0 ± 387.0 cells/mm^2 at 1 week (P = 0.0004) but increased back to baseline levels after 1 month (2424.0 ± 379.4 cells/mm^2, P = 0.3). This apparent reduction is endothelial cell count was most likely due to the attachment of inflammatory cell on the endothelium or a microscopic cellular edema separating the endothelial cells from the Descemet's membrane making them appear as dark areas of the specular microscopy impairing the accuracy of cell measurement. But by 1 month, when the inflammation and edema subsides, the cell counts were back to pre-treatment values. The incidence of corneal edema was reported to be around 0.8% after SLT.[96] White et al. similarly reported in a series of 10 patients that received 180° SLT treatment that subtle endothelial changes were noticeable on slit lamp examination but by 6 weeks, these changes disappeared.[100] SLT has been demonstrated to be safe even on corneal grafts after penetrating keratoplasty.[101] However, in a recent randomized control trial comparing the use of SLT versus prostaglandin analogue in Chinese patients with PACG with at least 180° of angle opening after laser iridotomy, the 6-month endothelial cell count was found to be 4.8% lower than the baseline (P = 0.001).[102] Differences to Lee et al.'s reported transient reduction of 4.5% could be attributed to the differences in angle configuration between the 2 populations. While Lee et al.'s population had open-angles, Narayanaswamy et al.'s population had PACG, and therefore the cornea was of a closer proximity to the trabecular meshwork making it more susceptible to the heat and energy of SLT.

In Lee et al.'s study, the CCT decreased by 1.1% from a baseline of 549.4 ± 37.6 to 543.9 ± 40.2 μm at 1 week post-SLT (P = 0.02) but returned to the baseline level by 1 month (P = 0.2). It has been postulated that heat dissipation to the corneal stroma could have resulted in a temporary thermal contraction of the collagen fibers, similar to what has been reported for the holmium YAG laser.[103] As the replenishing of keratocytes takes place, the CCT resumes back to normal thickness without clinical evidence of scarring. The spherical equivalent was statistically static before and after baseline although the 1-month visual acuity did improve after SLT treatment (from 0.3 LogMAR to 0.2 LogMAR), possibly due to subjective variations in visual acuity testing or the subjective association of SLT with a refractive laser surgery.[99]

On the whole for SLT in OAG, the cornea, inflammatory, and IOP changes following SLT seem to be mild and transient without any evidence of documented permanent changes on objective measurements. Patients with narrow angle configurations undergoing treatment should be made aware of the potential risks and complications to the cornea due to its close proximity to the area of treatment.

7

Effect of SLT on IOP Fluctuation

IOP is still the single most important modifiable risk factors for glaucoma progression even in NTG.[60, 104] IOP fluctuation may be a significant factor in glaucoma progression.[67, 105] Office hour IOP measurements do not reflect the effects of circadian rhythm and nocturnal posturing on IOP.[106] We have established in the previous chapters the efficacy of SLT for IOP reduction but what about in terms of IOP fluctuation? Kóthy *et al.*[107] found reductions in the 24-hour IOP fluctuation after SLT but Nagar *et al.*[57] reported that SLT's control of diurnal IOP variation was inferior prostaglandin analogues. Inter-visit IOP fluctuations have also been reported to be dampened following a 360° SLT treatment as compared to 180° SLT treatment.[42] In the past, the majority of studies involving IOP fluctuations required patients to be admitted overnight with IOP sampling taken every few hours apart.

A more recent technology that has been used to investigate the pattern of IOP-related fluctuations over a 24-hour period is the SENSIMED Triggerfish® (Sensimed AG, Lausanne, Switzerland). This wireless silicon contact lens sensor (CLS) measures the biodimensional changes over the corneoscleral junction, for 30 seconds every 5 minutes, collecting more than 300 data points during each interval. These points are then plotted on a graph repressing the IOP-related pattern. At present, the CLS records outputs in milli-volts equivalent (mVeq) rather than the clinically used mmHg thus, only the fluctuations from baseline can be compared. The device is a safe and tolerated method of measuring the 24-hour IOP-related pattern since the patient can sleep in the supine position with the CLS in-situ, without having to wake the patient up for IOP measurements at night unlike in conventional practices.[108, 109]

Lee et al.[110] used the CLS to investigate the IOP-related fluctuations in a group of 18 NTG subjects that underwent SLT. CLS recording was performed for 24-hours before and at 1 month after a single episode of SLT. The number and type of anti-glaucoma medications were kept constant in between these 2 periods. A cosine function was fitted to the mean CLS patterns to analyze the global variability for each subject with further segregations into a success and non-success group, where success was defined as ≥ 20% IOP reduction after SLT. Local variability from the mean curve was also studied at the diurnal, nocturnal, and 24-hour periods.

Eight patients (44%) had success with SLT and their cosine fitted (global) amplitude was reduced by 24.6%. In contrast, in the remaining subjects that was unsuccessful with SLT, their global amplitude increase of 19.2%, mainly driven by a 34.1% higher diurnal and a 21.9% higher 24-hour local variability. In those with success to SLT, there was no change in the local variability during the diurnal, nocturnal or 24-hour periods. The local variability is a reflection of the variation of raw CLS data points around the smoothed curve while the global variability is more representative of IOP-related fluctuation over 24 hours (Figures 2 A, B).

Nagar et al. [57] reported a 41% IOP reduction in 50% of SLT treated POAG or OHT subjects but in their study, IOP was only measured 4 times at 08:00, 11:00, 14:00 and 18:00 hours. A broader spectrum of IOP measurement is important. Kothy et al.[107] reported in a population of 26 POAG subjects that none had a mean IOP reduction of ≥ 20% when IOP was measured from 08:00 to 00:00 hours.

The debate on whether or not SLT affects the diurnal or nocturnal IOP fluctuation is still ongoing most likely as a result of the differences in anti-glaucoma medications used. Kothy et al.[107] reported 4 to 5 mmHg IOP fluctuation during the diurnal period after a 4-week washout of mediations before SLT. On the other hand, Lee et al.[111] found that in their medically treated POAG population, IOP range was only reduced in the nocturnal period. Both of these studies however, did not measure IOP in a continuous manner.

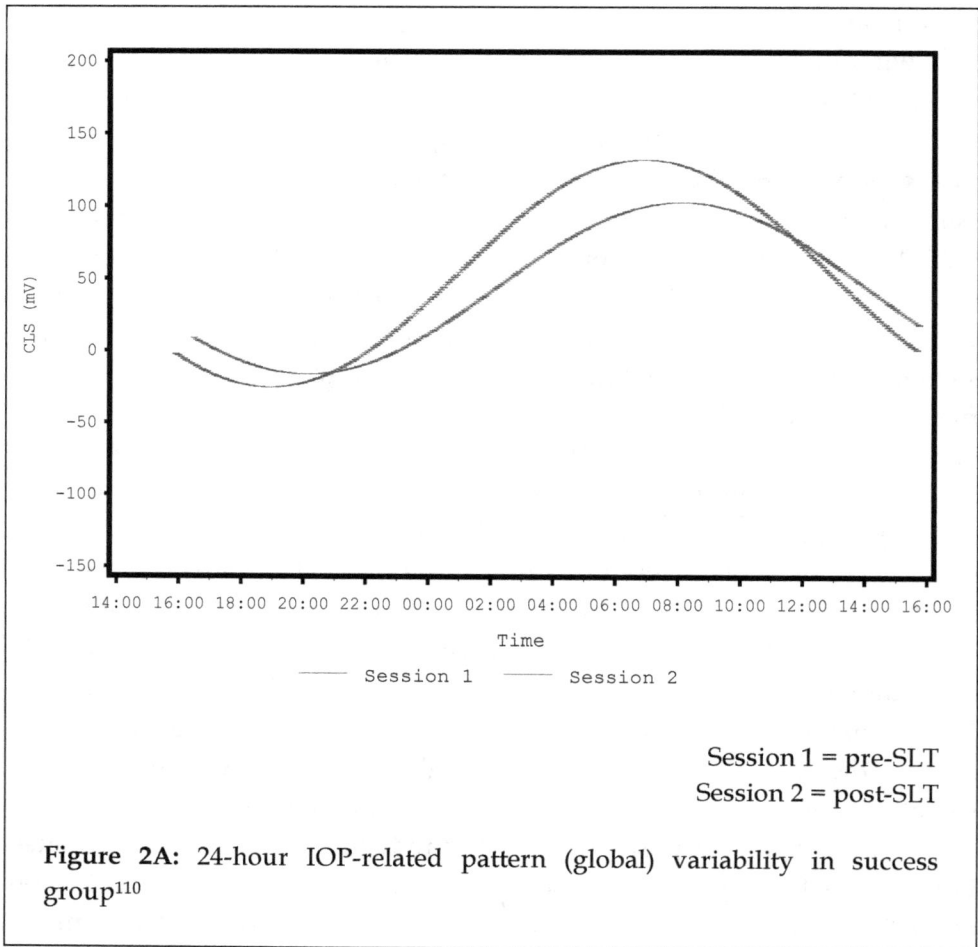

Figure 2A: 24-hour IOP-related pattern (global) variability in success group[110]

It seems that in those that success to SLT, they have also benefit from a reduction in their 24-hour IOP-related pattern fluctuation while those that did not respond to SLT seems to have a greater IOP-related pattern fluctuation especially during the daytime, which may be related to the wearing off of the evening dose of prostaglandin analogues which tend to reach peak effect at 8 – 12 hours after use.[112] Larger, prospective and randomized trials are needed to deepen our understanding on the influences of SLT on IOP fluctuation and disease progression.

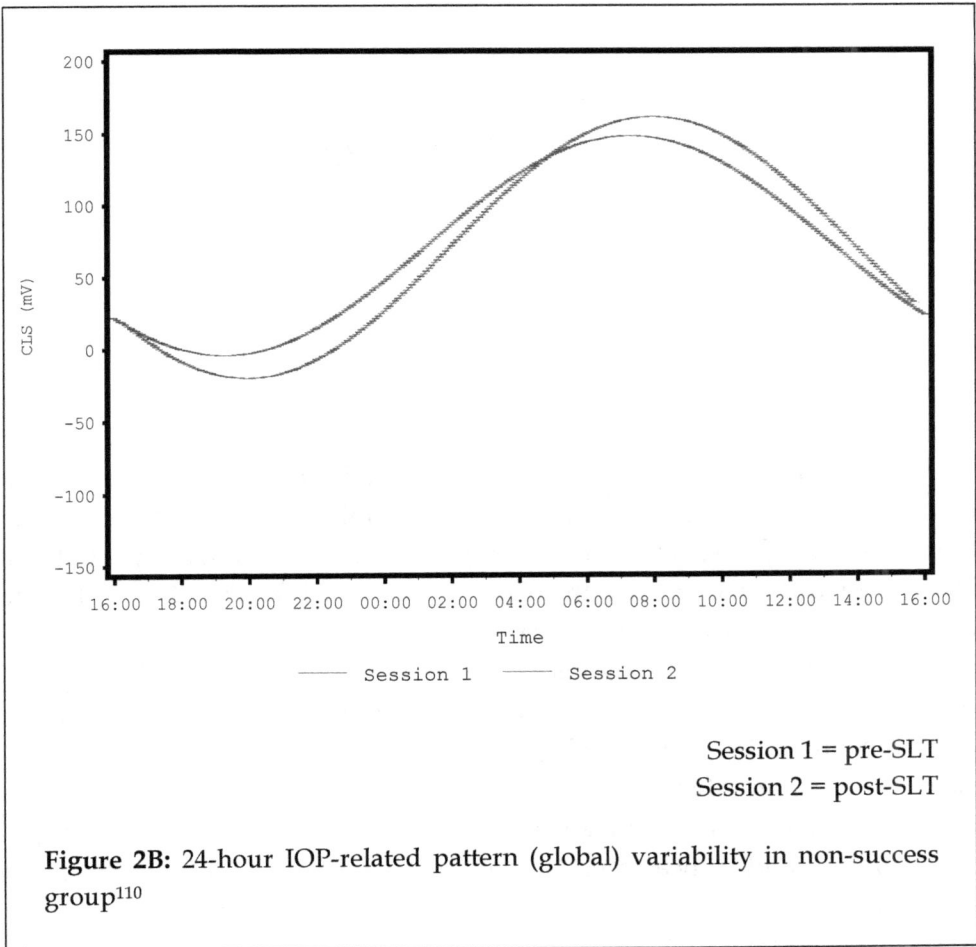

Figure 2B: 24-hour IOP-related pattern (global) variability in non-success group[110]

8

Effect of SLT on Quality of life

So far, the efficacy of SLT in reducing IOP, IOP fluctuations, and medications as well as its safety and predictability has been discussed in the earlier chapters. The Early Manifest Glaucoma Trial reported an absence of difference in health-related quality of life (HRQOL) between patients treated with a topical beta-blocker plus ALT versus no treatment in patients with newly diagnosed POAG.[113] Likewise, the Collaborative Initial Glaucoma Treatment Study also demonstrated no significant difference in quality of life (QOL) between those receiving medical versus surgical treatment for newly diagnosed POAG patients.[114] As SLT is effective in reducing the medication requirements, almost free of major side effects, and repeatable, the quality of life of patients may be improved.[23]

Lee et al.[62] investigated the effects of adjuvant SLT in a Chinese population of POAG subjects. Forty-one POAG subjects were randomized to continue topical anti-glaucoma medications versus receiving an adjuvant 360° SLT treatment. In both groups, medication was titrated to maintain a 25% reduction from the presenting IOP or an IOP of < 18 mmHg, whichever was lower. The translated Chinese versions of the Glaucoma Quality of Life - 15 (GQL-15) and a simplified Comparison of Ophthalmic Medications for Tolerability (COMTOL) survey scores were used to assess for QOL outcome.

The GQL-15 questionnaire is a glaucoma-specific questionnaire assessing patient's subjective difficulty in performing 15 daily tasks that are categorized into 4 major areas: 1) central and near vision, 2) peripheral vision, 3) dark adaptation and glare, and 4) outdoor mobility:

1.   Reading newspapers

2.   Walking after dark

3.   Seeing at night

4.   Walking on uneven ground

5.   Adjusting to bright lights

6.   Adjusting to dim lights

7.   Going from light to dark room or vice versa

8.   Tripping over objects

9.   Seeing objects coming from the side

10.   Crossing the road

11.   Walking on steps/stairs

12.   Bumping into objects

13.   Judging distance of foot to step/curb

14.   Finding dropped objects

15.   Recognizing faces

Each of the 15 items above are then given a subscale score from 1 to 5 depending on the level of perceived difficulty with 1 being the easiest and 5 being the most difficult. Zero is denoted if the patient does not perform the tasks involved for non-visual reasons. A higher score signifies a poorer quality of life.

The COMTOL questionnaire is a consistent, reliable, and reproducible assessment of the eye drop side effects.[115-117] A simplified version of the COMTOL was used in Lee *et al.*'s study, in a checklist style to see if subjects experienced any of the 15 local side effects, with a higher score representing greater intolerability to eye drops:

1.   Burning

2.   Blurred vision

3.   Tearing

4.   Itchy eyes

5.   Dimming of vision

6.   Discharge from eyes

7.   Focusing

8.   Reading

9.   Redness

10.   Bitter taste

11.   Swelling

12.   Dry eyes

13.   Troubles seeing at night

14.   Unusual taste

15.   Brow-ache

In both treatment arms, the baseline IOP, number of medication used, and baseline QOL scores were statistically similar. At 6 months, the SLT group had a 7.6% lower IOP (P = 0.03) and used 40.0% fewer medications (P = 0.02) compared to the medication group. And when compared with baseline, the SLT group also used fewer medications after the procedure (P < 0.0001). However, at 6 months, there was no statistically significant difference in the GQL-15 or COMTOL scores between the 2 treatment arms (P ≥ 0.2) as well as compared to the baseline (P ≥ 0.4) values in each arm respectively.

The absence of significant differences in QOL may be related to the design and limitation of the current QOL questionnaires available for glaucoma patients. There are 18 different glaucoma-specific patient-reported QOL surveys available and the GQL-15 is already one of the more favourable ones in terms of its content, validity, and reliability.[118] However, as the questionnaire only focuses on 4 areas that mainly revolve around changes in vision, it is unlikely these assessment parameters will change in a SLT patient in the short-term. In contrast, the practical benefits of SLT including medication reduction, convenience away from polypharmacy or IOP reductions, simply cannot be reflected from the questionnaire. Despite these shortcomings, we know from the literature that topical anti-glaucoma medications does affect treatment satisfaction and QOL due to the side effects of medications including burning sensation, blurring, and tearing.[117] The preservative, banzalkonium chloride, can also cause results in ocular surface disease in up to 59% of glaucoma patients receiving medical treatment.[119] The COMTOL checklist is one that shows consistency (0.73 to 0.98), reliability (0.76 to 0.94), and reproducibility (0.75 to 0.93) in the quantification of eye drop adverse effects.[115] The COMTOL score was reduced by 11.9% from baseline in the SLT treatment patients but increased by 2.2% from baseline in the medical group, although these changes were short of statistical significance.

While a single session of adjuvant SLT reduced IOP and medications, there were no detectable differences in QOL as compared to those using medication alone. This could be due to limitations in the design of the current glaucoma QOL surveys as well the need for longer-term studies to reflect QOL changes.

9

Future Developments in Laser Trabeculoplasty

Laser trabeculoplasty has evolved clinically and technologically over the years. There has been a shift from ALT to the newer SLT amongst clinicians, partly for its ease of use and theoretical repeatability and lower side effect profile. However, overall trabeculoplasty has fallen out of favor in recent years due to a number of factors. One of the factors is the introduction of highly efficacious topical medications, the recognition that the effects of trabeculoplasty are known to decline over time and in an unpredictable manner, potentially leaving patients uncontrolled between clinic visits. Thirdly, minimally invasive glaucoma surgeries, often combined with phacoemulsification, are gaining popularity and compete with trabeculoplasty for a very similar target population of OHT or mild to moderate OAG.

Despite all these challenges, trabeculoplasty still has a significant role in the management of glaucoma. New research is changing the treatment paradigm of SLT. Primary SLT, that is applying SLT before commencing medical therapy, was found to be more cost effective than glaucoma eye drops.[120, 121] Annual repeated SLT appears to be an effective and safe method to maintain IOP control and prevent IOP control drop off.[122] Although Lee *et al.* did not find any difference in QOL responses between SLT and medication, there is still evidence that patients value the convenience and comfort of being drop-free.[62] There are ongoing studies being conducted in the United Kingdom and Australia looking at the health related QOL in patients having initial SLT versus conventional medical therapy that will further our understanding of this area.

There are several new procedures that also modulate the TM, with the aim of increasing efficacy and/or lowering adverse reactions. These include MicroPulse Laser Trabeculoplasty (MLT), Titanium Sapphire Laser Trabeculoplasty (TSLT) and Pattern Scanning Laser Trabeculoplasty (PLT).

9.1   MicroPulse Laser Trabeculoplasty

MLT delivers energy in repetitive microsecond pulses. This allows energy to be delivered with intermittent cooling periods therefore reducing thermal build up and subsequent tissue damage.[123] Earlier studies used a 810 nm wavelength laser (similar to SLT) but later researchers have switched to 532 nm. MLT is thought to work by stimulating a biological response via cytokine release increasing aqueous outflow while reducing tissue damage.

Typical settings for MLT are 300 μm spot size (smaller than the 400 μm SLT spot size), 300 ms duration, 1000 mW power, 15% duty cycle, over 360° of the TM.[124, 125] The duty cycle indicates the percentage of time the laser will be active for the duration chosen. Radcliffe recommends 100 shots over 360° whereas Ahmed recommends confluent applications. There is no visible blanching or bubbles seen during the treatment process.[124, 125]

In a randomized pilot study comparing MLT to ALT in 21 eyes, both groups achieved around a 20% reduction of IOP at 3 months with no significant difference between the groups. This group used a laser setting of 300 μm spot size, 2000 mW energy, 200 ms duration, 15% duty cycle with 66 laser spots over the nasal 180°[126]. In a phase II prospective interventional case series, assessing 20 patients, MLT achieved a mean IOP reduction of around 20% at 12 months in 15 patients with a success rate of 75%. Five patients (25%) failed, 4 in the first week and 1 at 6 months. Only 1 patient had an IOP and anterior chamber flare that normalized after 3 days. The authors treated the inferior 180° using a 810 nm wavelength laser, 200 μm spot size, 2000 mW power, 200 ms duration with a 15% duty cycle and 70 – 84 laser spots.[127].

However, there is one published study that questions the efficacy of the MLT. A retrospective study of 40 patients with a mean follow up of 12 months, found only 1 patient (2.5%) had 20% or more reduction in IOP and 3 patients (7.5%) had ≥ 3 mmHg decrease in IOP at 19 months. The average time for failure was around 3 months. This study population had a relatively lower pre-treatment mean IOP of 21.8 ± 4.9 mmHg (range 14 – 34 mmHg) on a mean of 2 ± 1.3 medications. Laser settings used were: 300 µm spot size, 2000 mW power, 200 ms duration, 15% duty cycle, and 60 – 66 laser spots in 180° of the TM. [128]

There is currently an ongoing multi-center trial in North America assessing the efficacy of MLT. The preliminary data of 50 patients showed a reduction in IOP over 6 months with minimal-to-no IOP spikes and low inflammatory response.[124] The preliminary data of a study comparing MLT to SLT showed that the 2 technologies were comparable. Twelve eyes had MLT and 14 eyes had SLT. The mean IOP change was 3.9 mmHg versus 2.6 mmHg respectively.[129].

In one of the larger MLT series involving a Chinese population by Lee *et al.* in Hong Kong, 48 Chinese subjects with OAG were treated with a single session of MLT using a 577 nm MLT laser of 3 ms duration, 1000 mW energy, 15% duty cycle, and 120.5 ± 2.0 shots. At 6 months, the IOP was reduced by 19.5% and the number of medications was reduced by 21.4% with a response rate of 72.9%. Only 7.5% had a mild, self-limiting anterior uveitis that occurred between 1 to 4 weeks post-laser. [130]

The advantages of MLT become more apparent in patients at higher risk of post trabeculoplasty pressure spikes, such as highly pigmented trabecular meshwork. There have also been reports of success of MLT after previous SLT[131]. MLT has shown encouraging responses in these early studies. The hope is that MLT can prove to be a safer version of SLT but with equal efficacy.

9.2   Titanium Sapphire Laser Trabeculoplasty

TSLT uses a longer wavelength (790 nm) than either SLT or the current MLT technologies. This near-infrared wavelength is thought to allow deeper penetration to the juxtacanalicular meshwork and selective absorption by pigmented phagocytic cells, preserving TM tissue.[132] There is very limited published clinical data on TSLT and the product is not widely available. A study published in 2009 compared TSLT to ALT in 37 patients. The TSLT group had an 8 mmHg (32%) reduction in mean IOP compared to the ALT group, which had a 6.5 mmHg (25%) reduction. There was no statistical difference between the 2 groups The number of medications decreased from 1.4 ± 1.0 to 1.3 ± 1.0 in the TSLT group and from 2.1 ± 0.8 to 2.0 ± 0.8 in the ALT group and IOP spikes occurred in 1 of the patients that received TSLT and 3 of the patients who underwent ALT. No peripheral anterior synechiae formation was noted in the TSLT eyes, but it was not an uncommon occurrence in the ALT eyes.[132] A larger unpublished study compared TSLT with ALT in 175 patients. Eighty-five patients received TSLT and 89 patients underwent ALT for POAG. The results largely confirmed those of the previously mentioned research.[133]

9.3   Pattern Scanning Trabeculoplasty

PLT utilizes the computer-guided technology of the PASCAL (Topcon Europe Medical BV, ssebaan 11, 2908 LJCapelle aan den IJssel, The Netherlands) laser to apply multiple, short duration laser applications in a segment pattern to the TM It is a continuous wave light with a wavelength of 532 nm. The suggested settings are: 100 μm spot size, 5 – 10 ms duration and a titrated power to achieve tissue blanching. Each treatment pattern consists of 2 or 3 rows (24 to 36 spots) of arching spots that correspond to 22.5° of trabecular meshwork angle. Eight adjacent treatment segments corresponds to 180° of the TM and 16 treatment segments equates to 360°. It is thought to create less tissue injury compared to ALT due to its much shorter pulse durations reducing the thermal injury diffusion distance. The efficacy is maintained by applying approximately 10 times more spots.[134]

In a prospective study, 47 eyes in 25 patients were treated with 360° of PLT, in 16 treatment segments. Each segment consisted of 66 spots arranged in 3 rows. Spot size of 100 μm and power titrated until TM blanching at 10 ms duration. Once the power is titrated, the duration was reduced to 5 ms. The authors also developed a computer-guided pattern scanning algorithm. After the completion of each segment, the aiming beam automatically rotates 22.5° to that the user then rotates the gonioscopy treatment lens to apply the laser to the next segment. The average IOP decrease was from 21.9 ± 4.1mmHg to 15.5 ± 2.7 mmHg at 6 months of follow up. However, 17 eyes were excluded from the 6 months data due to either a viral conjunctivitis or requiring additional IOP-lowering therapy. Twenty of the 30 eyes (67%) had an IOP drop of more than 20% (definition of success) with an average IOP reduction of 24%. There were no pressure spikes or inflammation reported. [134]

There are 2 published studies comparing ALT to PLT. In a German study, PLT showed a reduction of mean IOP from 20.2 ± 1.1 to 15.6 ± 0.8 mmHg (P < 0.001) in 20 eyes of 20 patients at around 8 weeks of follow up. There was no statistical difference in the reduction in IOP compared to ALT (P = 0.26).[135] In a second study from Korea, PLT had a mean IOP reduction of 27.1%, from 24.1 ± 4.2 mmHg to 17.6 ± 2.6 mmHg (P = 0.03) at 6 months and again showed no statistical difference to ALT.[136]

MLT, TSLT and PLT are promising new technologies with the goal of making trabeculoplasty safer and more effective. Further studies will be needed to determine if these challengers can replace SLT as the standard trabeculoplasty treatment.

References

1. Giaconi JA. Laser Trabeculoplasty: ALT vs SLT. (20 January 2015). Retreived from URL: http://eyewiki.aao.org/Laser_Trabeculoplasty %3A_ALT_vs_SLT.

2. Zweng HC, Flocks M. Experimental photocoagulation of the anterior chamber angle. A preliminary report. Am J Ophthalmol 1961;52:163-5.

3. Krasnov MM. Laseropuncture of anterior chamber angle in glaucoma. Am J Ophthalmol 1973;75(4):674-8.

4. Worthen DM, Wickham MG. Argon laser trabeculotomy. Trans Am Acad Ophthalmol Otolaryngol 1974;78(2):OP371-5.

5. Wise JB, Witter SL. Argon laser therapy for open-angle glaucoma. A pilot study. Arch Ophthalmol 1979;97(2):319-22.

6. The Glaucoma Laser Trial Research Group. The Glaucoma Laser Trial (GLT). 2. Results of argon laser trabeculoplasty versus topical medicines. The Glaucoma Laser Trial Research Group. Ophthalmology 1990;97(11):1403-13.

7. Kramer TR, Noecker RJ. Comparison of the morphologic changes after selective laser trabeculoplasty and argon laser trabeculoplasty in human eye bank eyes. Ophthalmology 2001;108(4):773-9.

8. Latina MA, Park C. Selective targeting of trabecular meshwork cells: in vitro studies of pulsed and CW laser interactions. Exp Eye Res 1995;60(4):359-71.

9.   Latina MA, Sibayan SA, Shin DH, *et al.* Q-switched 532-nm Nd:YAG laser trabeculoplasty (selective laser trabeculoplasty): a multicenter, pilot, clinical study. Ophthalmology 1998;105(11):2082-8; discussion 9-90.

10. Stein JD, Challa P. Mechanisms of action and efficacy of argon laser trabeculoplasty and selective laser trabeculoplasty. Curr Opin Ophthalmol 2007;18(2):140-5.

11. Melamed S, Pei J, Epstein DL. Delayed response to argon laser trabeculoplasty in monkeys. Morphological and morphometric analysis. Arch Ophthalmol 1986;104(7):1078-83.

12. van der Zypen E, Fankhauser F. Ultrastructural changes of the trabecular meshwork of the monkey (Macaca speciosa) following irradiation with argon laser light. Graefes Arch Clin Exp Ophthalmol 1984;221(6):249-61.

13. Van Buskirk EM, Pond V, Rosenquist RC, Acott TS. Argon laser trabeculoplasty. Studies of mechanism of action. Ophthalmology 1984;91(9):1005-10.

14. Samples JR, Alexander JP, Acott TS. Regulation of the levels of human trabecular matrix metalloproteinases and inhibitor by interleukin-1 and dexamethasone. Invest Ophthalmol Vis Sci 1993;34(12):3386-95.

15. Bradley JM, Anderssohn AM, Colvis CM, *et al.* Mediation of laser trabeculoplasty-induced matrix metalloproteinase expression by IL-1beta and TNFalpha. Invest Ophthalmol Vis Sci 2000;41(2):422-30.

16. Bylsma SS, Samples JR, Acott TS, Van Buskirk EM. Trabecular cell division after argon laser trabeculoplasty. Arch Ophthalmol 1988; 106(4):544-7.

17. Acott TS, Samples JR, Bradley JM, *et al.* Trabecular repopulation by anterior trabecular meshwork cells after laser trabeculoplasty. Am J Ophthalmol 1989;107(1):1-6.

18. Narayanaswamy A, Leung CK, Istiantoro DV, *et al.* Efficacy of selective laser trabeculoplasty in primary angle-closure glaucoma: a randomized clinical trial. JAMA Ophthalmol 2015;133(2):206-12.

19.   Ho CL, Lai JS, Aquino MV, *et al*. Selective laser trabeculoplasty for primary angle closure with persistently elevated intraocular pressure after iridotomy. J Glaucoma 2009;18(7):563-6.

20.   Abdelrahman AM, Eltanamly RM. Selective laser trabeculoplasty in Egyptian patients with primary open-angle glaucoma. Middle East Afr J Ophthalmol 2012;19(3):299-303.

21.   Babighian S, Caretti L, Tavolato M, *et al*. Excimer laser trabeculotomy vs 180 degrees selective laser trabeculoplasty in primary open-angle glaucoma. A 2-year randomized, controlled trial. Eye (Lond) 2010; 24(4):632-8.

22.   Birt CM. Selective laser trabeculoplasty retreatment after prior argon laser trabeculoplasty: 1-year results. Can J Ophthalmol 2007;42(5): 715-9.

23.   Bovell AM, Damji KF, Hodge WG, *et al*. Long term effects on the lowering of intraocular pressure: selective laser or argon laser trabeculoplasty? Can J Ophthalmol 2011;46(5):408-13.

24.   Cvenkel B. One-year follow-up of selective laser trabeculoplasty in open-angle glaucoma. Ophthalmologica 2004;218(1):20-5.

25.   El Mallah MK, Walsh MM, Stinnett SS, Asrani SG. Selective laser trabeculoplasty reduces mean IOP and IOP variation in normal tension glaucoma patients. Clin Ophthalmol 2010;4:889-93.

26.   Goldenfeld M, Geyer O, Segev E, *et al*. Selective laser trabeculoplasty in uncontrolled pseudoexfoliation glaucoma. Ophthalmic Surg Lasers Imaging 2011;42(5):390-3.

27.   Gracner T. Intraocular pressure reduction after selective laser trabeculoplasty in primary open angle glaucoma. Coll Antropol 2001;25 Suppl:111-5.

28.   Gracner T. Intraocular pressure response of capsular glaucoma and primary open-angle glaucoma to selective Nd:YAG laser trabeculoplasty: a prospective, comparative clinical trial. Eur J Ophthalmol 2002;12(4):287-92.

29.   Hirneiss C, Sekura K, Brandlhuber U, *et al.* Corneal biomechanics predict the outcome of selective laser trabeculoplasty in medically uncontrolled glaucoma. Graefes Arch Clin Exp Ophthalmol 2013.

30.   Hu YD, Chen L. Effect of selective laser trabeculoplasty on ocular hypertension. [Chinese]. International Journal of Ophthalmology 2009;9(5):879-81.

31.   Juzych MS, Chopra V, Banitt MR, *et al.* Comparison of long-term outcomes of selective laser trabeculoplasty versus argon laser trabeculoplasty in open-angle glaucoma. Ophthalmology 2004; 111(10):1853-9.

32.   Kara N, Altan C, Satana B, *et al.* Comparison of selective laser trabeculoplasty success in patients treated with either prostaglandin or timolol/dorzolamide fixed combination. J Ocul Pharmacol Ther 2011;27(4):339-42.

33.   Katz LJ, Steinmann WC, Kabir A, *et al.* Selective laser trabeculoplasty versus medical therapy as initial treatment of glaucoma: a prospective, randomized trial. J Glaucoma 2012;21(7):460-8.

34.   Koucheki B, Hashemi H. Selective laser trabeculoplasty in the treatment of open-angle glaucoma. J Glaucoma 2012;21(1):65-70.

35.   Kulkami A, Goyal S, O'Brart D. Comparison of Low and High Power Selective Laser Trabeculoplasty in Ocular Hypertension and Primary OpenAngle Glaucoma. American Academy of Ophthalmology2008.

36.   Lai JS, Chua JK, Tham CC, Lam DS. Five-year follow up of selective laser trabeculoplasty in Chinese eyes. Clin Experiment Ophthalmol 2004;32(4):368-72.

37.   Liu Y, Birt CM. Argon versus selective laser trabeculoplasty in younger patients: 2-year results. J Glaucoma 2012;21(2):112-5.

38.   Maeda S, Konno S, Oguchi S, Ohtsuka K. Long-term outcome of selective laser trabeculoplasty as correlated with circadian intraocular pressure. [Japanese]. Japanese Journal of Clinical Ophthalmology 2006;60(5):781-5.

39.   Mahdy MA. Efficacy and safety of selective laser trabeculoplasty as a primary procedure for controlling intraocular pressure in primary

open angle glaucoma and ocular hypertensive patients. Sultan Qaboos Univ Med J 2008;8(1):53-8.

40. Melamed S, Ben Simon GJ, Levkovitch-Verbin H. Selective laser trabeculoplasty as primary treatment for open-angle glaucoma: a prospective, nonrandomized pilot study. Arch Ophthalmol 2003; 121(7):957-60.

41. Nitta K, Sugiyama K, Mawatari Y, Tanahashi T. Results of selective laser trabeculoplasty (SLT) as initial treatment for normal tension glaucoma. Nihon Ganka Gakkai Zasshi 2013;117(4):335-43.

42. Prasad N, Murthy S, Dagianis JJ, Latina MA. A comparison of the intervisit intraocular pressure fluctuation after 180 and 360 degrees of selective laser trabeculoplasty (SLT) as a primary therapy in primary open angle glaucoma and ocular hypertension. J Glaucoma 2009;18(2):157-60.

43. Qian SH, Sun XH. Selective laser trabeculoplasty in the treatment of primary open-angle glaucoma. Zhonghua Yi Xue Za Zhi 2007;87(2): 118-20.

44. Rosenfeld E, Shemesh G, Kurtz S. The efficacy of selective laser trabeculoplasty versus argon laser trabeculoplasty in pseudophakic glaucoma patients. Clin Ophthalmol 2012;6:1935-40.

45. Seymenoglu G, Baser EF. Efficacy of Selective Laser Trabeculoplasty in Phakic and Pseudophakic Eyes. J Glaucoma 2013.

46. Shazly TA, Smith J, Latina MA. Long-term safety and efficacy of selective laser trabeculoplasty as primary therapy for the treatment of pseudoexfoliation glaucoma compared with primary open-angle glaucoma. Clin Ophthalmol 2010;5:5-10.

47. Song J, Lee PP, Epstein DL, et al. High failure rate associated with 180 degrees selective laser trabeculoplasty. J Glaucoma 2005;14(5): 400-8.

48. Tang M, Fu Y, Fu MS, et al. The efficacy of low-energy selective laser trabeculoplasty. Ophthalmic Surg Lasers Imaging 2011;42(1):59-63.

49. Thatsnarong D, Ngamchittiampai C, Phoksunthorn T. One year results of selective laser trabeculoplasty in the treatment of primary open angle glaucoma. J Med Assoc Thai 2010;93(2):211-4.

50. Tokuda N, Inoue J, Yamazaki I, *et al.* Effects of selective laser trabeculoplasty treatment in steroid-induced glaucoma. Nihon Ganka Gakkai Zasshi 2012;116(8):751-7.

51. Tzimis V, Tze L, Ganesh J, *et al.* Laser trabeculoplasty: an investigation into factors that might influence outcomes. Can J Ophthalmol 2011;46(4):305-9.

52. Vyborny P, Sicakova S. Selective laser trabeculoplasty--new possibilities in glaucoma treatment. Cesk Slov Oftalmol 2009;65(1): 8-11.

53. Werner M, Smith MF, Doyle JW. Selective laser trabeculoplasty in phakic and pseudophakic eyes. Ophthalmic Surg Lasers Imaging 2007;38(3):182-8.

54. Russo V, Barone A, Cosma A, *et al.* Selective laser trabeculoplasty versus argon laser trabeculoplasty in patients with uncontrolled open-angle glaucoma. Eur J Ophthalmol 2009;19(3):429-34.

55. Kent SS, Hutnik CM, Birt CM, *et al.* A Randomized Clinical Trial of Selective Laser Trabeculoplasty Versus Argon Laser Trabeculoplasty in Patients With Pseudoexfoliation. J Glaucoma 2013.

56. Wong MO, Lee JW, Choy BN, *et al.* Systematic review and meta-analysis on the efficacy of selective laser trabeculoplasty in open-angle glaucoma. Surv Ophthalmol 2014.

57. Nagar M, Luhishi E, Shah N. Intraocular pressure control and fluctuation: the effect of treatment with selective laser trabeculoplasty. Br J Ophthalmol 2009;93(4):497-501.

58. Nagar M, Ogunyomade A, O'Brart DP, *et al.* A randomised, prospective study comparing selective laser trabeculoplasty with latanoprost for the control of intraocular pressure in ocular hypertension and open angle glaucoma. Br J Ophthalmol 2005;89(11):1413-7.

59. Gray TA, Orton LC, Henson D, *et al*. Interventions for improving adherence to ocular hypotensive therapy. Cochrane Database Syst Rev 2009(2):CD006132.

60. Heijl A, Leske MC, Bengtsson B, *et al*. Reduction of intraocular pressure and glaucoma progression: results from the Early Manifest Glaucoma Trial. Arch Ophthalmol 2002;120(10):1268-79.

61. The Advanced Glaucoma Intervention Study (AGIS): 7. The relationship between control of intraocular pressure and visual field deterioration.The AGIS Investigators. Am J Ophthalmol 2000;130(4): 429-40.

62. Lee JW, Chan CW, Wong MO, *et al*. A randomized control trial to evaluate the effect of adjuvant selective laser trabeculoplasty versus medication alone in primary open-angle glaucoma: preliminary results. Clin Ophthalmol 2014;8:1987-92.

63. Sturmer J, Meier-Gibbons F. The diagnosis of normal-tension glaucoma. Curr Opin Ophthalmol 1994;5(2):64-8.

64. Iwase A, Suzuki Y, Araie M, *et al*. The prevalence of primary open-angle glaucoma in Japanese: the Tajimi Study. Ophthalmology 2004;111(9):1641-8.

65. Kim CS, Seong GJ, Lee NH, Song KC. Prevalence of primary open-angle glaucoma in central South Korea the Namil study. Ophthalmology 2011;118(6):1024-30.

66. Comparison of glaucomatous progression between untreated patients with normal-tension glaucoma and patients with therapeutically reduced intraocular pressures. Collaborative Normal-Tension Glaucoma Study Group. Am J Ophthalmol 1998;126(4):487-97.

67. Collaer N, Zeyen T, Caprioli J. Sequential office pressure measurements in the management of glaucoma. J Glaucoma 2005;14(3):196-200.

68. Schwartz AL, Perman KI, Whitten M. Argon laser trabeculoplasty in progressive low-tension glaucoma. Ann Ophthalmol 1984;16(6):560-2, 6.

69. Best UP, Domack H, Schmidt V. Long-term results after selective laser trabeculoplasty - a clinical study on 269 eyes. Klin Monbl Augenheilkd 2005;222(4):326-31.

70. Hirn C, Zweifel SA, Toteberg-Harms M, Funk J. Effectiveness of selective laser trabeculoplasty in patients with insufficient control of intraocular pressure despite maximum tolerated medical therapy. Ophthalmologe 2012;109(7):683-90.

71. Lee JW, Ho WL, Chan JC, Lai JS. Efficacy of selective laser trabeculoplasty for normal tension glaucoma: 1 year results. BMC Ophthalmol 2015;15(1):1.

72. Lee JW, Gangwani RA, Chan JC, Lai JS. Prospective study on the efficacy of treating normal tension glaucoma with a single session of selective laser trabeculoplasty. J Glaucoma 2015;24(1):77-80.

73. Lee JW, Shum JJ, Chan JC, Lai JS. Two-Year Clinical Results After Selective Laser Trabeculoplasty for Normal Tension Glaucoma. Medicine (Baltimore) 2015;94(24):e984.

74. Brooks AM, Grant G, Gillies WE. Reversible corneal endothelial cell changes in diseases of the anterior segment. Aust N Z J Ophthalmol 1987;15(4):283-9.

75. Scherer WJ. Effect of topical prostaglandin analog use on outcome following selective laser trabeculoplasty. J Ocul Pharmacol Ther 2007;23(5):503-12.

76. Alvarado JA, Iguchi R, Juster R, et al. From the bedside to the bench and back again: predicting and improving the outcomes of SLT glaucoma therapy. Trans Am Ophthalmol Soc 2009;107:167-81.

77. Singh D, Coote MA, O'Hare F, et al. Topical prostaglandin analogues do not affect selective laser trabeculoplasty outcomes. Eye (Lond) 2009;23(12):2194-9.

78. Ayala M, Chen E. Predictive factors of success in selective laser trabeculoplasty (SLT) treatment. Clinical Ophthalmology 2011;5(1):573-6.

79. Barkana Y, Belkin M. Selective laser trabeculoplasty. Surv Ophthalmol 2007;52(6):634-54.

80. George MK, Emerson JW, Cheema SA, *et al.* Evaluation of a modified protocol for selective laser trabeculoplasty. J Glaucoma 2008;17(3): 197-202.

81. Lee JW, Wong MO, Liu CC, Lai JS. Optimal Selective Laser Trabeculoplasty Energy for Maximal Intraocular Pressure Reduction in Open-Angle Glaucoma. J Glaucoma 2015.

82. Lee JW, Chan JC, Chang RT, *et al.* Corneal changes after a single session of selective laser trabeculoplasty for open-angle glaucoma. Eye (Lond) 2013.

83. Johnson PB, Katz LJ, Rhee DJ. Selective laser trabeculoplasty: predictive value of early intraocular pressure measurements for success at 3 months. Br J Ophthalmol 2006;90(6):741-3.

84. Rachmiel R, Trope GE, Chipman ML, *et al.* Laser trabeculoplasty trends with the introduction of new medical treatments and selective laser trabeculoplasty. J Glaucoma 2006;15(4):306-9.

85. Kano K, Kuwayama Y, Mizoue S, Ito N. Clinical results of selective laser trabeculoplasty. Nihon Ganka Gakkai Zasshi 1999;103(8):612-6.

86. Martow E, Hutnik CM, Mao A. SLT and adjunctive medical therapy: a prediction rule analysis. J Glaucoma 2011;20(4):266-70.

87. Lee JW, Liu CC, Chan J, *et al.* Predictors of success in selective laser trabeculoplasty for primary open angle glaucoma in Chinese. Clin Ophthalmol 2014;8:1787-91.

88. Lee JW, Liu CC, Chan JC, Lai JS. Predictors of success in selective laser trabeculoplasty for chinese open-angle glaucoma. J Glaucoma 2014;23(5):321-5.

89. Lee JW, Liu CC, Chan JC, Lai JS. Predictors of success in selective laser trabeculoplasty for normal tension glaucoma. Medicine (Baltimore) 2014;93(28):e236.

90. Kim YJ, Moon CS. One-year follow-up of laser trabeculoplasty using Q-switched frequency-doubled Nd:YAG laser of 523 nm wavelength. Ophthalmic Surg Lasers 2000;31(5):394-9.

91. Traverso CE, Spaeth GL, Starita RJ, *et al*. Factors affecting the results of argon laser trabeculoplasty in open-angle glaucoma. Ophthalmic Surg 1986;17(9):554-9.

92. Schwartz AL, Whitten ME, Bleiman B, Martin D. Argon laser trabecular surgery in uncontrolled phakic open angle glaucoma. Ophthalmology 1981;88(3):203-12.

93. Hodge WG, Damji KF, Rock W, *et al*. Baseline IOP predicts selective laser trabeculoplasty success at 1 year post-treatment: results from a randomised clinical trial. Br J Ophthalmol 2005;89(9):1157-60.

94. Mao AJ, Pan XJ, McIlraith I, *et al*. Development of a prediction rule to estimate the probability of acceptable intraocular pressure reduction after selective laser trabeculoplasty in open-angle glaucoma and ocular hypertension. J Glaucoma 2008;17(6):449-54.

95. Latina MA, de Leon JM. Selective laser trabeculoplasty. Ophthalmol Clin North Am 2005;18(3):409-19, vi.

96. Latina MA, Tumbocon JA. Selective laser trabeculoplasty: a new treatment option for open angle glaucoma. Curr Opin Ophthalmol 2002;13(2):94-6.

97. Moubayed SP, Hamid M, Choremis J, Li G. An unusual finding of corneal edema complicating selective laser trabeculoplasty. Can J Ophthalmol 2009;44(3):337-8.

98. Regina M, Bunya VY, Orlin SE, Ansari H. Corneal edema and haze after selective laser trabeculoplasty. J Glaucoma 2011;20(5):327-9.

99. Lee JW, Chan JC, Chang RT, *et al*. Corneal changes after a single session of selective laser trabeculoplasty for open-angle glaucoma. Eye (Lond) 2014;28(1):47-52.

100. White AJ, Mukherjee A, Hanspal I, *et al*. Acute transient corneal endothelial changes following selective laser trabeculoplasty. Clin Experiment Ophthalmol 2012.

101. Nakakura S, Imamura H, Nakamura T. Selective laser trabeculoplasty for glaucoma after penetrating keratoplasty. Optom Vis Sci 2009;86(4):e404-6.

102. Narayanaswamy A, Leung CK, Istiantoro DV, *et al.* Efficacy of Selective Laser Trabeculoplasty in Primary Angle-Closure Glaucoma: A Randomized Clinical Trial. JAMA Ophthalmol 2014.

103. Tanaka T, Furutani-Miura S, Nakamura M, Nishida T. Immuno-histochemical study of localization of extracellular matrix after holmium YAG laser irradiation in rat cornea. Jpn J Ophthalmol 2000;44(5):482-8.

104. The effectiveness of intraocular pressure reduction in the treatment of normal-tension glaucoma. Collaborative Normal-Tension Glaucoma Study Group. Am J Ophthalmol 1998;126(4):498-505.

105. Asrani S, Zeimer R, Wilensky J, *et al.* Large diurnal fluctuations in intraocular pressure are an independent risk factor in patients with glaucoma. J Glaucoma 2000;9(2):134-42.

106. Barkana Y, Anis S, Liebmann J, *et al.* Clinical utility of intraocular pressure monitoring outside of normal office hours in patients with glaucoma. Arch Ophthalmol 2006;124(6):793-7.

107. Kothy P, Toth M, Hollo G. Influence of selective laser trabeculoplasty on 24-hour diurnal intraocular pressure fluctuation in primary open-angle glaucoma: a pilot study. Ophthalmic Surg Lasers Imaging 2010;41(3):342-7.

108. Lorenz K, Korb C, Herzog N, *et al.* Tolerability of 24-hour intraocular pressure monitoring of a pressure-sensitive contact lens. J Glaucoma 2013;22(4):311-6.

109. Mansouri K, Medeiros FA, Tafreshi A, Weinreb RN. Continuous 24-hour monitoring of intraocular pressure patterns with a contact lens sensor: safety, tolerability, and reproducibility in patients with glaucoma. Arch Ophthalmol 2012;130(12):1534-9.

110. Lee JW, Fu L, Chan JC, Lai JS. Twenty-four-hour intraocular pressure related changes following adjuvant selective laser trabeculoplasty for normal tension glaucoma. Medicine (Baltimore) 2014;93(27):e238.

111. Lee AC, Mosaed S, Weinreb RN, *et al.* Effect of laser trabeculoplasty on nocturnal intraocular pressure in medically treated glaucoma patients. Ophthalmology 2007;114(4):666-70.

112. Russo A, Riva I, Pizzolante T, *et al.* Latanoprost ophthalmic solution in the treatment of open angle glaucoma or raised intraocular pressure: a review. Clin Ophthalmol 2008;2(4):897-905.

113. Heijl A, Bengtsson B, Hyman L, Leske MC. Natural history of open-angle glaucoma. Ophthalmology 2009;116(12):2271-6.

114. Janz NK, Wren PA, Lichter PR, *et al.* Quality of life in newly diagnosed glaucoma patients : The Collaborative Initial Glaucoma Treatment Study. Ophthalmology 2001;108(5):887-97; discussion 98.

115. Barber BL, Strahlman ER, Laibovitz R, *et al.* Validation of a questionnaire for comparing the tolerability of ophthalmic medications. Ophthalmology 1997;104(2):334-42.

116. Beckers HJ, Schouten JS, Webers CA, *et al.* Side effects of commonly used glaucoma medications: comparison of tolerability, chance of discontinuation, and patient satisfaction. Graefes Arch Clin Exp Ophthalmol 2008;246(10):1485-90.

117. Nordmann JP, Auzanneau N, Ricard S, Berdeaux G. Vision related quality of life and topical glaucoma treatment side effects. Health Qual Life Outcomes 2003;1:75.

118. Vandenbroeck S, De Geest S, Zeyen T, *et al.* Patient-reported outcomes (PRO's) in glaucoma: a systematic review. Eye (Lond) 2011;25(5):555-77.

119. Skalicky SE, Goldberg I, McCluskey P. Ocular surface disease and quality of life in patients with glaucoma. Am J Ophthalmol 2012;153(1):1-9 e2.

120. Lee R, Hutnik CM. Projected cost comparison of selective laser trabeculoplasty versus glaucoma medication in the Ontario Health Insurance Plan. Can J Ophthalmol 2006;41(4):449-56.

121. Seider MI, Keenan JD, Han Y. Cost of selective laser trabeculoplasty vs topical medications for glaucoma. Arch Ophthalmol 2012;130(4): 529-30.

122. Gandolfi S, Ungaro N. Low power selective laser trabecuoplasty (slt) repeated yearly as primary treatment in ocular hypertension: long

term comparison with conventional slt and alt. Arvo 2014 Annual Meeting. Orlando, USA2014.

123. Vujosevic S, Bottega E, Casciano M, *et al.* Microperimetry and fundus autofluorescence in diabetic macular edema: subthreshold micropulse diode laser versus modified early treatment diabetic retinopathy study laser photocoagulation. Retina 2010;30(6):908-16.

124. Ahmed IK. Excellent Safety Profile of MicroPulse Laser Trabeculoplasty (MLT) for Glaucoma. Glaucoma Today 2014; November/December 2014.

125. Radcliffe NM. MLT offers safe, well-tolerated approach to lower IOP, reduce need for medication. OphthalmologyTimes 2014.

126. Ingvoldstad DD, Krishna R, Willoughby L. Micropulse Diode Laser Trabeculoplasty versus Argon Laser Trabeculoplasty in the treatment of Open Angle Glaucoma. ARVO 2005.

127. Fea AM, Bosone A, Rolle T, *et al.* Micropulse diode laser trabeculoplasty (MDLT): A phase II clinical study with 12 months follow-up. Clin Ophthalmol 2008;2(2):247-52.

128. Rantala E, Valimaki J. Micropulse diode laser trabeculoplasty -- 180-degree treatment. Acta Ophthalmol 2012;90(5):441-4.

129. Coombs P, Radcliffe NM. Outcomes of Micropulse Laser Trabeculoplasty vs. Selective Laser Trabeculoplasty. ARVO2014.

130. Lee JW, Yau GS, Yick DW, Yuen CY. MicroPulse Laser Trabeculoplasty for the Treatment of Open-Angle Glaucoma. Medicine (Baltimore) 2015;94(49):e2075.

131. Tai T. Micropulse Laser Trabeculoplasty After Previous Laser Trabeculoplasty. Glaucoma Today2014; V. November/December 2014.

132. Goldenfeld M, Melamed S, Simon G, Ben Simon GJ. Titanium:sapphire laser trabeculoplasty versus argon laser trabeculoplasty in patients with open-angle glaucoma. Ophthalmic Surg Lasers Imaging 2009;40(3):264-9.

133. Reiss GR. The titanium sapphire laser opens a new frontier. Glaucoma today 2012(march/april):27-8.

134. Turati M, Gil-Carrasco F, Morales A, *et al.* Patterned laser trabeculoplasty. Ophthalmic Surg Lasers Imaging 2010;41(5):538-45.

135. Barbu CE, Rasche W, Wiedemann P, *et al.* Pattern laser trabeculoplasty and argon laser trabeculoplasty for treatment of glaucoma. Ophthalmologe 2014;111(10):948-53.

136. Kim JM, Cho KJ, Kyung SE, Chang MH. Short-Term Clinical Outcomes of Laser Trabeculoplasty Using a 577-nm Wavelength Laser. J Korean Ophthalmol Soc 2014;55(4):563-9.